How

# My FREE Gift

Dear Reader,

I want to give you a personal gift. With this present I hope I can contribute to your well-being so you may live a healthier, better quality life.

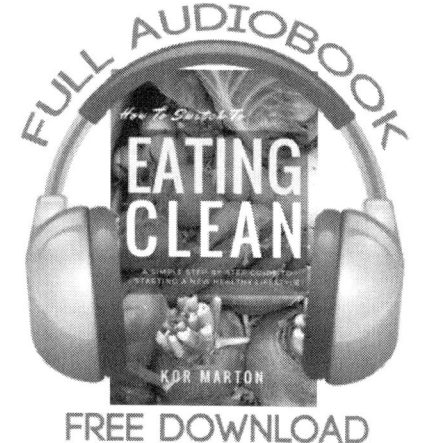

This is the URL to download your copy of the FULL FREE AUDIO BOOK: http://eatingclean.kormarton.com/
Please make sure you put in your best email address when asked, as I will email the secret download link directly to you.
If you like my free audio book, leave a review and let me know!

I hope with this free gift I can give you great value and provide some support for your healthy endeavors.
Thank You for giving it a chance!

Stay Healthy My Friend!


Kor Marton

How To Switch To Eating Clean

# IN OPENING

## About The Author

Kor Marton is a prime example of a self-started, self-taught, self-made weight loss coach. What started out only as a hobby turned into his full time passion and ultimately, his track records as a nutritionist show that, being a healthy nutrition evangelist is his true calling in this world.

According to his own admission, by the age of 45, he is in the best shape of his life both physically and mentally, therefore welcomes every challenge and feels unstoppable on every level. Frankly, it shows: he is more successful than ever but it hasn't always been this way.

As a young artist-entrepreneur he did the usual "bad stuff" every young man would when trying to live life to the fullest: partying, drinking and even experimenting with recreational drugs of all sorts.

He started struggling with being more and more overweight in his late twenties. By his early thirties he was able to clean up his act as a drinker, smoker and drug user but still grossly overweight so he ventured out to find the perfect weight loss diet that would make him weigh «normal», again.

After being fed up with an unbroken chain of unsuccessful fad diets he realized it wasn't an actual «magic pill» or «secret formula» or some other weight loss innuendo that he needed: it was a total shift in his nutritional consciousness. He needed a new lifestyle that could be just as enjoyable as sustainable.

During the past fifteen years Kor went through the bulk of mainstream and alternative nutritional science literature, gathering and assembling all relevant information regarding general nutrition, well-being and weight management.

He is down to earth, full of positive energies, he can inspire you and be inspired by you.
In short, he is just like you - except he knows a lot about weight management.
Please listen to him when he talks, read his books when he writes. I do, too.

**Noémi Staha**
Author, Nutritionist

## Who Am I?

That is a great question! After all, why should you listen to me if you don't even know who I am?
Then let me introduce myself: My name is Kor Marton. I was born in Hungary about 45 years ago. I spent the first half of my life in Hungary and I was fortunate enough to spend the other half in Los Angeles, California. It was there where the «health bug» bit me.

I am an autodidact nutritionist or a self-taught dietician, if you prefer the latter term. I also happen to be a very active man (some would even say I am a fitness enthusiast). So these factors along with being very passionate about wanting to help others achieve what I have achieved made me realize: lately I am becoming somewhat of a healthy lifestyle guru on the internet. Nevertheless, I am just a simple man with simple pleasures.

I started my «journey» towards healthy living a long time ago. Yes, I am old. I must have been in my early thirties. I was younger yet I was always fat, tired, depressed and sick. I didn't actually have a medical condition but I never felt as horrible as back then. I knew something needed to be done.

I started researching. 15 years ago the internet was still a joke so I took advantage of my free library membership and huge selection of healthy nutrition books at the Beverly Hills Public Library. Yes, I am talking about physical, dusty, heavy paper books! (Kids these days don't even know how good they have it!)

As a result of my early findings I started eating cleaner and behold - I started feeling, looking, performing in my life better! The funny thing was that I started my journey weighing 220 lbs (which is about 100 kg in metric) and I am now weighing the same!

## How To Switch To Eating Clean

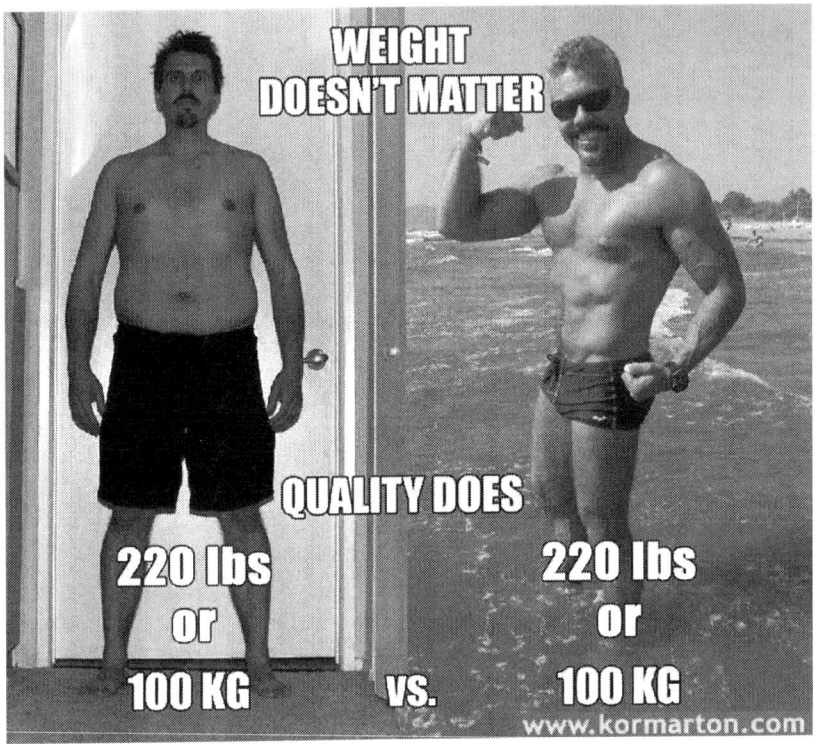

«What changed then?» - you might ask. Quality did. My body fat was about 33% back then and it is only about 10% these days. But it is not just that I have less body fat: I also have more lean muscle, a super-fast metabolism, a strong immune system and my bone structure is strong, too. So it seems weight loss is not a very accurate expression. Maybe we should talk about losing body fat instead of losing weight...

# How To Switch To Eating Clean

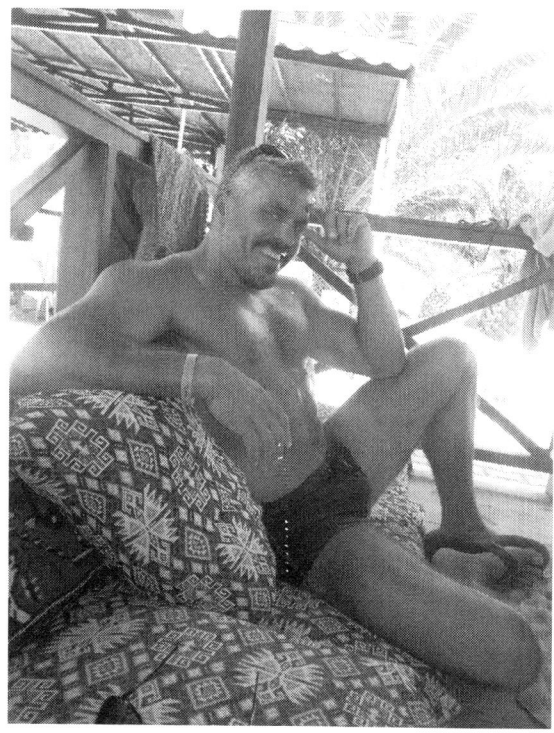

They say information is power. And it is so true. My story could be a true testament that an everyday guy like me in his forties can achieve a strong, lean body and a superior level of health just by obtaining and applying the right information. Thanks to the intelligent and informal persuasion of world famous nutritionist Noémi Staha I am currently a «veganish-vegetarianish» clean eater, never looked/felt/performed better in my life but my research today is still an on-going project. Which I enjoy with a passion.

In this book I would like to share with you my findings that were responsible my effortless transitioning from eating crappy to eating clean.
I truly hope it will help you at least as much as it did help me!

## Preface

This book is intended to those who decided to make a major improvement in their lives and could use some guidance in switching to eating clean.
This book is also perfect for those who are only considering the switch and curious whether they could do it or how much of a strain it would put on them. (Not much - I can tell you upfront but we will address this later.)
Important: This is not a recipe book!
It is a lot more than that!
You probably know the saying give a man a fish and you feed him for a day; teach a man to fish and you feed him for a lifetime.
Well, this book intends to do exactly just that: teach you the concept of eating clean!
If you want recipes please buy my 365 Days of Eating Clean Recipes cookbook because this book is a collection of carefully selected information and will guide you through the principles of eating clean and not the meals themselves. It will give you a lot of valuable information which you will need as you take your first steps in the direction of healthy living.
Some pieces of information may be something you might have already known, some will be brand new to you, hopefully.
If you have this book, you really don't need recipes. Once you become familiar with the concept of eating clean, even some of your old, «not-so-clean» recipes could be revised and «made clean» based on the principles gathered here.
Either way, I would like to congratulate you for your decision of embarking on this wonderful and exciting journey and getting this book as your first sign of dedication!

## How To Switch To Eating Clean

With the information this book contains, I would really like to make an impact, a difference in the world however small it might be.

My motto has always been and always will be: «Making the world a healthier place - one person at a time.»

# EATING CLEAN

# How To Switch To Eating Clean

# What Is Eating Clean?

There are many definitions but I think the most accurate one is this: eating clean is eating real, whole, unprocessed foods, as close to their natural state as possible, most of the time.

When you eat clean you choose to eat vegetables, fruits, high quality carbs like sweet potatoes, whole grains, good quality proteins mostly from plant sources, healthy fats and oils, like avocados, nuts, cold pressed oils like extra virgin olive oils, etc.

When you decide to eat clean you need to realize that it is not a "temporary thing" like a weight loss or fad diet; it is a lifestyle choice and it is meant to be a long term one.

One of the main ideas behind eating clean is that you are making conscious efforts to be in charge of your own physical and mental health, energy levels and general well-being.

This way, you can avoid the cravings, mood-swings and all the other unwanted side effects of eating low quality, nutrient void foods that leave us hungry most of the time. Of course, these symptoms may look, feel and be different for everyone, nevertheless, they exist when you don't eat clean.

Eating clean itself may also mean a different diet for everyone. A vegetarian will eat clean differently than, say, a vegan or a meat-eater or an athlete. It is not just the kinds of foods that may differ for each but also the amounts, the daily number of meals and even the methods of preparation or the spices used.

The only hard rule here, again, is that you eat real, whole, unprocessed foods, as close to their natural state as possible most of the time, with one more possibly important addendum: which you love eating. It makes total sense when you think about it: if you don't love eating clean it will hardly work out for you as a chosen lifestyle.

## What Are Highly Processed Foods?

When we talk about highly processed foods we talk about the ones that go through multiple stages of heavy processing before they end up in front of you, on your dining table. These foods usually come in bags or boxes and made in factories so we might as well call them factory foods.

"Why are highly processed foods so bad?" - you might ask. Great question! One of the major side effects of food processing is that the nutrients which are naturally present in most foods are being destroyed by every pass of processing. This also means if there are less nutrients in your food less nutrient will go into your body and I hope you start seeing the problem with that.
A great way of identifying a food as highly processed is by looking at the list of ingredients on the food label. If it is a long list with weird or sometimes even "chemistry class" sounding names chances are that the food you are looking at is highly processed.

Another huge problem with highly processed foods is that they are engineered to hit that "evolutionary" spot by overloading them with sugars, fats and salt. These can lead to a strongly euphoric state shortly after consuming them because these ingredients, mainly in refined forms, may trigger a heavy dopamine release by the reward center of your brain. People who eat highly processed foods on a regular basis usually don't have a problem with this because they feel what they eat is very satisfying.

## How To Switch To Eating Clean

The last thing which needs to be mentioned is possibly the worst of the food additives a.k.a. the taste bud killers: the flavor enhancers. As our body is a biochemical power plant some of our functions can be easily manipulated by chemicals. When you taste actual real tastes it is also chemicals acting, the only difference is in the strength.

Flavor enhancers are able to chemically mimic the taste of something that "tastes good" but with a strength so overwhelming that your tastebuds become desensitized to real flavors. No wonder, whoever eats a lot of highly processed foods probably eats a lot of flavor enhancers so they are physically (or should I say chemically) incapable of enjoying the subtleties in flavor of real foods, making them hardly ever want to eat anything other than what actually «hits the spot»: processed foods. Once you know about this weird biochemical illusion it is but obvious why clean eating gets a bad reputation from processed food eaters claiming that «it doesn't taste good» - but now at least you know why this is.

Similarly, when after a loud concert your hearing is so desensitized due to the blaring music that once you are out of the arena, you can barely hear your buddy talking next to you.

In a weird experiment scientists swept up the dirt from the lab floor and sprinkled it with some flavor enhancer. They were curious whether the lab rats would like it or not. Just so you understand, I am talking about non-edible stuff spiked with some flavor enhancer being fed to laboratory animals. Once again, dirt swept up from the lab floor. Yes, a mixture of dust, hairs and other gross miscellaneous microscopic items. Can you guess what happened? The lab rats ate it up in a frenzy like it was cake. This should tell you all.

## How To Switch To Eating Clean

# Five Main Guidelines For Your Transition

### 1. Start Cooking As Often As You Can!
This is possibly the easiest way to start your journey towards eating clean! When you cook you have full control over everything from ingredients through freshness, preparation methods down to the smallest details like spices or preferred way of serving.

### 2. Read Your Food Labels!
When you start doing this, if you haven't already been doing it, you will start to gain an understanding of what is actually going into your body with your food. Now, I don't say all food labels are telling us the whole truth and nothing but the truth, but they legally don't have much wiggle room for fibbing (depending on where you live, of course) so it is a good start.
A great rule of thumb is to try sticking with foods that have five or less ingredients, which ingredients you either know, recognize or at least you can pronounce.

### 3. Avoid Highly Processed Foods At All Cost
Industrial food processing has different processing levels. Most foods that we know as health foods might be slightly processed. For example, like most cashews, quinoa or even oatmeal is slightly processed. This doesn't mean that you need to stay away from these foods but always choose the ones with the least amount of processing, whenever you have the choice.

If you are only embarking on your journey towards clean eating just recently, I highly recommend making baby steps and focusing on the worst stuff at first: no frozen pizzas, no Twinkies, no hot pockets, no TV Dinners. Later, you may want to raise your standards by cutting out more, maybe not so highly but still badly processed foods so your general food choices really get cleaner and cleaner with time. Only do this if you introduce alternatives to those you cut out and you understand that the cleaner you will eat the better your natural flavoring skills need to be. This is a also a great opportunity for you to get to like not just amazing new dishes but also exciting new flavors. I think you catch my drift...

## 4. Avoid Artificial Flavors and Sweeteners
I have to make a strong point: artificial flavors and sweeteners are NOT real food! Again, we are dealing with a factory made food product that was specifically designed to bypass your brain's logical part and only tickle the pleasure points in the reward center of your brain. Recreational drugs are engineered similarly. No wonder you want more and more of it and don't even understand why!

Admittedly, this «wanting more» has two parts:
The psychological part: "This is (calorie free, sugar free, low calorie, etc. - insert your term here) so I can have more of it because it doesn't count!"
And then there's the physical part: It tricks your body into craving more sweets, so good luck resisting. It will make you get fat long term.

Your body actually has no idea what to do with the artificial chemicals once they are inside - which on its own can be a huge health hazard.

While it is mostly highly processed foods which contain artificial stuff of all sorts, they are not the only ones! Think of drinks, dressings, spice mixes, in some countries even salt has added artificial chemicals!

## 5. Watch Your Macronutrient Balance
Macronutrients are the carbohydrates, proteins and fats you consume. These are the elemental building blocks of your diet. I don't recommend going too crazy about counting them, at least not at first, but a general daily

## How To Switch To Eating Clean

macronutrient awareness is strongly advised, mainly when you are just getting started.

Interestingly, carbs from processed foods add up faster while, at the same time, we may not get enough heart healthy fats into our system.

When, during your day, you eat more clean foods that are rich in good quality macronutrients you will feel fuller, stay full longer, have more energy because your body starts functioning better on every level.

Once again: baby steps! Little changes regarding the quality of your macronutrient balance, tiny shifts in your eating habit towards the clean direction will have a significant impact on your body and your health.

The goal here is to create a well balanced system of meals for most days by understanding the actual impact of the food choices you make.

## How To Switch To Eating Clean

# Love What You Eat!

This is probably the most important message to anyone wanting to switch to eating clean! Just a friendly reminder: if it is a lifestyle choice you will be "stuck" with it so might as well enjoy it! Many people do so it is not at all impossible although pushing away from the commercially available food products can be a serious challenge these days.

Cooking (or food preparation) is not just a great way to have control over what goes into your food and into your body! It is a crazy good opportunity to "build a relationship" with the food you eat.
It starts with where you get it from, through how you prepare it and ends with how it tastes and feels in your belly.

As weird as it sounds, studies have shown if you make your own food you will like it more. Mostly when you get really good at making your food and become a Jedi of using spices just the way you like them. May the salt be with you!

Remember, if you want clean eating to be your lifestyle it has got to be sustainable so first of all, enjoy the process! If you look at making or preparing your own food as some sort of obstacle you will have a lot of stress and frustration which clearly defeats the original purpose.
In other words, try to find the path that will lead you to where you want to be but the path must be a happy and enjoyable one!

## Prerequisites

This is a list of things I find important but not necessarily vital for your success. Ideally, it would be best to have a touch of everything so you can start working on them. Please don't panic, if you don't have some of them or only have partial ones. This is just for your awareness so you may or may not want to or have to work on them.

**Your WHY**
Just like for any good success story, possibly the most important prerequisite for you to have is a very strong WHY.
WHY do you want to eat clean? The answer may make it or break it.
Your WHY will determine the drive behind your actions, the wind under your wings or the fire under your butt. Your WHY can be anything that is something you either would like to reach or stay away from.

I know a clean eater whose WHY is health related: he has been diagnosed with early onset type 2 diabetes and wanted to do something about it, the natural way.
I know some others who eat clean because they are hobby performance athletes, just to mention two extremes.
In my first example, the WHY is a frightening medical condition from which the person involved wants to stay away.
In the second one, the WHY is the desire to perform better and winning some local championships is the motivation.
These two WHY, from the opposite end of the spectrum, can be equally strong driving forces but ultimately each of them are very personal.
So here's my advice: find your very personal WHY and you will find success!

# How To Switch To Eating Clean

**Supporting Environment**
It is easy to make tiny changes or even big ones when you live by yourself or with roommates who buy their own food, separate from you or have a family which fully supports your choices, not just with words but with actions, too. Now let's think of the ones who are not in such fortunate situations! They may have a family which may not be supportive enough and either tease, mock or openly laugh at the person who is trying implement some healthy changes in their own life.

Some other issues may rise from the logistical nightmare of regularly having to prepare two kinds of foods: traditional or processed food for one part of the family and clean foods for the other. This can also be a problem if the person making the switch is or was a heavy highly processed food eater and may still be battling the demons of basic withdrawals. It really doesn't matter that you are fully aware how bad highly processed foods are or how much you love your new clean food lifestyle; if temptation is there with you in a weak moment, your journey may slow down or ultimately even end due to the number of bad food choices you start making.

If you are dealing with the lack of a supporting environment and you are not in the position to change it, try to turn the odds in your favor by focusing on your personal WHY.

**Good Logistics And Organizing Skills**
When you have been eating clean for a while you already know where you can get your good, quality food and it may come from different places. When you start out at first, a trip to the supermarket may be satisfactory (also, greatly depending on the type and quality of your supermarket) but once you raise the bar and your standards get higher with time the supermarket may only become one of the stops you make because you will start picking up some of your food at farmers' markets, butchers or carnicerias.

## How To Switch To Eating Clean

This is where I need to mention that seasonal fruits and veggies are the bomb! True, they also require your seasonal attention. For example, when it is strawberry season eat strawberries while they are fresh! Also, buy way more than you can eat (let's say, a boatload of it - technical term!) and as a side project, you clean and bag them for your freezer. This, of course, can be done with mostly any fruits and veggies that you can freeze.

I am a seasoned clean eater and also a busy man. I used to go to the farmers' market myself until I ended up making some real good connections and I could strike up a deal with some of the open minded farmers there. To this day, some of the fruit and produce providers come to my home 2-4 times a week (but usually on a regular schedule) with a selection of bio-organic fruits and vegetables they already know I will like.

The other great thing about this is that I will never have the excuse of not having fresh, quality food at home and resort to eating subpar stuff.

Oh and I haven't even told you the best part! I actually pay less than what I would at the market because I am a regular customer and I technically almost buy bulk. Once again, I know my situation is not typical but clearly shows that a solution will always present itself as soon as you start looking for it.

## How To Switch To Eating Clean

# Preparations

There really no need to make any preparations unless you come from the far dark side of the highly processed food empire. Then, yes, maybe.

I am talking about those who have a very unhealthy relationship with highly processed foods or some of its ingredients like refined sugar.

Sugar addiction is a very unfortunate and widely occurring phenomena these days. It is not an epidemic but only because sugar addiction is not a disease, yet over 80% of Americans are addicted to sugar. Now this sounds like a huge number and it is really alarming although we need to take it into consideration that this number represents all sugar addicts of varying a degrees from light to heavy. The chance of being addicted and very similar statistics apply to flour and processed foods, as well.

Sugar addiction, mainly in its light form, often goes unrecognized so here are five clues that will help you determine whether you may be addicted to sugar, flour and processed food:

- You eat certain foods even if you are not hungry
- You eat certain foods only because you crave them
- You KNOW you should cut down on certain foods
- You often feel sluggish, fatigued or even exhausted due to overeating
- You have health issues or even social problems (affecting your everyday functions) because of your food choices yet you keep eating the way you do despite the obvious negative consequences
- You need more and more of the foods you crave to experience any pleasure or reduce negative emotions

If any of these apply to you you may want to be aware of it because then at least you know what you are dealing with.

## How To Switch To Eating Clean

Obviously, the more addicted you are the worse your sugar cravings will be, so this should be one of the first things you want to learn to control when embarking on your clean eating journey as a sugar addict.

Here are a few tips that will help you curb your sugar cravings:
Do NOT use artificial sweeteners!
Logic dictates that if you are addicted to sugar you want to stay away from it but substituting is not the right thing to do!
I already talked about artificial sweeteners in this book so even if repetition is the mother of learning I wouldn't want to be redundant about how it is engineered and how it tricks your brain into wanting more or even craving sugar. Once again, I can't help but try to be explicit enough and scream from the top of my lungs that artificial sweeteners are technically nerve poisons!! Aspartame, cyclamate, saccharin and many others fall into this category.
The false sense of security you may have regarding consuming them is only due to the slick marketing strategies that cost the giant multi-national food concerns billion dollars annually. So be aware and keep a watchful eye for food labels and ingredients!

The other reason I haven't yet mentioned is that most artificial sweeteners are a lot (about 200-400 times) sweeter than real sugar so imagine what they can do to your taste buds and palate! After consumption you will end up craving sweet stuff and so much, that even sugar wouldn't prove to be sweet enough for you! It is a surefire way to lose your sense of tasting real food real quick AND put on some excess fat if you can't resist your strong secondary cravings!

A great solution to cut down on artificial sweeteners is minimizing sugar altogether while switching to a better quality sugar source like honey, agave syrup or maple syrup and scale it down little by little, with time.

## How To Switch To Eating Clean

Ultimately these can also be totally eliminated by using various fruits but we will talk about that in another book.

### Sleep A Lot!
Your body is a lot smarter than you think! It knows that the fastest way to get energy for your body is from sugar. Did you notice that you usually start craving high carb foods like candy bars, chocolate, pasta or even bread when you feel sleepier? Like when the afternoon low hits? Well, now you know why! Guess what happens when you are not sleepy? That's right, your body doesn't want to wake itself up by energizing it with sugar!
The biggest favor you can do to yourself is to go to bed early and wake up early or take a short power nap when you feel you need one. This way you will have less sugar cravings due to sleepiness!

### Eat More Naturally Sweet Foods!
Your body needs sugar but all sugars were not created equal! Naturally sweet foods contain sugars but in quantities that is enough for you but not enough to make you fat, so your body gets what it needs in a much more subtle way. These sugars can only be absorbed in a timely manner. Why? Sugars in fruits and vegetables can be found mixed in between the fibers which act like biochemical timers so your body doesn't get all the sugars at once but little by little. This way your glycemic index doesn't go through the roof so insulin will not flood your bloodstream therefore excess fat doesn't even have a chance to be created.
A few good example for naturally sweet foods are sweet potatoes (and pretty much all root vegetables), pumpkins, brown rice, oatmeal and obviously most fibrous fruits.

### Check Your Protein Intake
Your body needs protein. The only thing is: too much or not enough protein can cause major sugar cravings. Now, this is where it gets personal! Handling this can get a little

## How To Switch To Eating Clean

tricky as you will have to figure out for yourself whether you eat too much, too little or just enough.

Here is a classic protein intake calculation algorithm for the person with the average body:

your body weight in lbs x 0.6 = grams of protein you need daily

Example:
You weigh 100 lbs so you need:
100 x 0.6 = 60g of protein daily

If you do heavy resistance training, like lifting weights or have some other fitness goals like gaining lean muscle this 0.6 could go up to as high as 1.0-1.2 so you will definitely need more protein.

**Know Your Real Habits**
Eating habits are not necessarily and directly linked to eating clean however it is a good practice to eliminate basic flaws in your eating habits so they don't stand in the way of your transitioning to eating clean.
Recent studies have shown that over 71% of people are not fully aware of their own eating habits or have discrepancies in major details between how they remember and actual reality when surveyed.
A significant number of people was not able to clearly identify the correct number of meals they actually consumed in a day, another significant number of the same target group was convinced they had consumed enough servings of vegetables when in fact they didn't and some of them did NOT even (!) consume any!

The best way to overcome this biased memory issue is to write your own food log for at least a few days. In this log, you write down your «input» and «output»: every time you eat, drink or go to the bathroom. Putting down approximate

## How To Switch To Eating Clean

amounts, qualities and time stamping them is also a good idea.

Looking at your food log after three days or so you will either see a pattern emerge or not see any patterns. If you do see a pattern it can indicate either good or bad eating habits (depending on the data) but the latter one means that your eating habits are closer to chaotic and you most likely need structure in your life.

One way to clearly identify how closely you eat to the recommended 70/30 ratio (consuming at least 70% plant based and not more than 30% animal based foods) is to highlight your food log using the following color coding:
highlight everything that is fruit or vegetables using a green highlighter
highlight everything that is animal based such as meats, eggs and dairy with a red highlighter
Highlight sugary carbohydrates using yellow
These «yellow» carbs are the following:
- sugars, honey, jams, fruit preserves
- pops and soft drinks, boxed juices
- potatoes, any shape or form of corn
- mueslis, (corn) flakes
- breads, pastries
- any forms of sweets and candies (like chocolate, candy bars, lollipops, pies, cakes, donuts, etc.), chips, (salted) pretzels, rice, all kinds of wheats, rye, oats, etc.

Once you are able to objectively identify the issues with your current eating habits it is a lot easier to find fixes.

### Easy Does It!
When you transition into eating clean it is advisable to do it slowly and very gradually. Actually, the slower the better. Any drastic change today maybe very costly tomorrow, mostly when you are not fully aware of the consequences of decisions regarding your food.

## How To Switch To Eating Clean

The basic principle is that a little change goes a long way and time along with consistency are much more important factors than the actual perfection of your present food quality.

Your choices should come little by little just so that you can make the transition as smoothly and unnoticeably as possible. Leaving the subpar food choices behind, or better yet, replacing them with more and more superior foods. This should be happening in a way that is not abrupt or doesn't pose even as a light trauma to your body or psyche. In other words, it should be a seamless transition where even you don't notice much as you go.

You may want to improve a little of your eating habits at a time, to erode your bad choices by a thousand tiny and almost imperceptible reductions and adding new dimensions of dietary choices millimeter by millimeter, inch by inch, at the same time.

It may also help you to keep focus on finding the good and appealing in your new choices (e.g.: how your newer foods taste better or make you feel more energized, etc.)

Remember, it took you years and years, possibly decades to develop your old, bad eating habits so go slow on the new ones but stay consistent!
Take your time, don't rush anything - easy does it!

Self education is also paramount as most people will not hire a nutritionist to think and strategize for them, instead of them. Reading books, listening to audiobooks, frequenting nutritional authority blogs, watching videos of the same on Youtube are just a few basic ways to get the knowledge you need in order to elevate yourself to higher levels of conscious, healthy nutrition.

# MAKING THE SWITCH

# Switch To Eating Clean: A Step-By-Step Guide

By now you should have a more thorough understanding of the basic principles of eating clean. Here is a step-by-step guide I recommend you to follow when you are ready to switch to a healthier gear in life. If done properly, this will make your transition to eating clean a lot easier and a lot less confusing.

## STEP 1 - CLEAN OUT YOUR FOOD RESERVES

This one is kind of self explanatory. You will need to go through all the places where you store/keep food: your fridge, your freezer, your pantry, your cabinets, cupboards and shelves.
This step has multiple sub-steps or individual tasks so you have the choice to do them all at once or step by step, depending on how quickly you want to switch to eating clean.

1. Start by tossing out everything that has expired.
You will be surprised how much crap you have that is no longer advisable to consume. Studies show that over 40% of people have at least one item that has expired months ago still sitting in their fridge or pantry!

2. The second part of your mission is to throw out everything that is heavily processed and/or has additives like preservatives, flavor enhancers or food coloring.
You can determine this by carefully reading the food labels. These items are usually the factory packaged, ready-to-eat foods.
Whether they are instant Ramen soups, canned stuff or frozen hot pockets - they've got to go!

## How To Switch To Eating Clean

If you are a meat eater and your meat products don't have labels because they are actually raw or grilled meat and not made in a factory, you may keep them. But ONLY keep the quality meats that ARE NOT PROCESSED! Most salamis, cold cuts, baloneys or hot dogs are full of additives and other harmful chemicals. Even the ones that your butcher slices up and custom-packages for you. Naturally, these won't have labels, but please assume they are chock full of these chemicals just the same and get rid of them!

3. Finally, throw out all the artificial sweetener containing and refined sugar laden foods! This includes not just the candy bars and chocolates but also soft drinks (both diet or regular) and, of course, sugar itself.

## STEP 2 - STOCK UP ON THE GOOD STUFF

Fill up your fridge with vegetables, fruits, quality dairy and other staple foods!
Whether you are an omnivore, vegetarian or vegan the following items should always be present in your fridge:

### **Water**
PROBABLY THE MOST IMPORTANT ITEM IN YOUR FRIDGE!!
Keep filtered or still mineral water in the refrigerator and you'll always have a cold, refreshing, healthy drink on hand. Zero water filter is one of the best filters there is and is a great way to get super healthy quality drinking water on demand!
For my recommendations on the best water filters for the lowest prices please visit my blog!
http://weightloss.kormarton.com/water-filter-recommendations/

## How To Switch To Eating Clean

I already did the legwork for you so all you have to do is look around there. You may also find more tips, tricks and suggestions regarding utensils and accessories for clean eating on my blog.

If you like your water with ice cubes make sure to buy ice made from filtered water, or make your own from the water you filter. Unless you efficiently filter your tap water, I do not recommend using your fridge's built in water filter. They are usually of low quality or just not good enough for human consumption...
Try using your ice cubes within two months if they are in a sealed bag or one month if not in a bag.

**Leafy greens and vegetables**
Bags of baby spinach, arugula and other leafy greens are a shopping-list staple! The pre-washed greens in single-variety bags last the longest. Always try going for the bio-organic or organic variety! Salad mixes are ok too if you eat them right away. They can become a problem if you don't use them in a day or two because they tend to spoil faster.

**Produce**
What most people don't seem to know: in most cases, produce should be kept out of the fridge entirely because most fridges, by default, are too cold for fruits and veggies. They should be kept cool but not quite «fridge cold». A dark, cool pantry is your best option but alternatively, you can keep them in the bottom bin of your fridge, where humidity can be controlled. When vegetables lose moisture, they get limp and may lose precious nutrients. This is because your fridge out-of-the-box is optimized for keeping food for omnivorous diets. As meats and dairy products need a lower cooling temperature.
Leafy greens, on the other hand, are usually better off in the bottom bin for the same reason: they can lose up to 50 percent of their vitamin C content along with their inside moisture if left out overnight.

# How To Switch To Eating Clean

### Oils
Extra virgin olive, cold pressed sunflower, and sesame oil are your healthiest options. If you have all three, you'll be able to cook just about anything. If you have a pantry store your oils in there, or in your fridge to keep them safe from heat and light. Spoiled (oxidized) oils do not just taste rancid they are also really bad for your health. Chilled oils may become cloudy, but they will quickly clarify at room temperature.

### Whole grains
Brown rice, whole-wheat flour, and oatmeal are the best grains to stock, but it is highly recommended to keep them cold. Refined grains, or better know as the «white ones», are white mostly because they are bleached and they also do not contain the most nutritious part of the grain: the outer bran and the inner seed, or germ.
Bleaching is a chemical process and even on its own is a good enough reason to drop white grains altogether.
The germ naturally contains some vegetable oil which can oxidize fairly quickly if not stored cold.
I also recommend stocking up on the not-so-well-known grains like buckwheat and quinoa.

### Sweet snacks
When frozen, berries and grapes end up tasting like cold gumdrops. Frozen sliced bananas become chewy and they can also be enjoyed as healthy snacks.
Blend frozen banana slices with spinach leaves, orange juice, berries, and maybe even yogurt (if you are not a vegan) for a yummy breakfast smoothie. If your fruits are frozen no ice is needed! Have a stronger blender or a wonderful Thermomix? Drop the juice (or even the yogurt) but add some more frozen fruits and you have yourself a killer, super healthy ice cream!
Either will give you satisfaction without giving you fat.

## How To Switch To Eating Clean

**Bananas**
When bananas become browned or just too spotted to pack them in your lunch box as snacks, throw them into your freezer. Make sure they are unpeeled! The skins may turn dark or even black, but the fruit will stay perfectly sweet and ripe inside. If you freeze them sliced you will want to eat them within a month or two.

**Nuts**
Chill or even freeze an assortment of almonds, cashews, hazelnuts and walnuts! They are naturally full of antioxidants and the fat in them are of the good kind! Nuts are mostly made up of monounsaturated fats which your body actually needs in order to function well. Just like oils, nuts too need to be kept cold and out of the light to remain fresh.

**Hummus**
Also known as garbanzo beans puree.
Always keep a little on hand. It is great for spreading and dipping too! Just add a bag of baby carrots and you get a combo which is a low-fat, high-protein snack alternative to hunks of cheese or a handful of cookies.

The following food items could also be staples if you are not a vegan:

**Cheese**
Replace mellow, soft cheeses with sharp, harder ones. A small amount packs lots of flavor, saving you both dollars and fat grams. Look for aged Cheddar and Parmigiano-Reggiano.

## How To Switch To Eating Clean

**Eggs**
Always buy farm raised, or free range chicken eggs. They may be smaller in size but usually pack a lot more nutrients.
Keep them on a lower shelf in your fridge and be sure to consume them within a week for maximum freshness.

**Butter and margarine**
Use real butter where it counts, but sparingly. Keep sticks in a covered dish. (Freeze sticks you're not using.) When it comes to margarine, I am not the biggest fan. I am sure you already guessed why; they are factory made «food products» but not real food.
The ones labeled "trans-fat free" are the only better butter substitutes but ultimately I recommend ditching margarine altogether.

**Milk, yogurt**
Fat free milk is neither healthy nor it is easy to cook with so if you are a milk drinker get the low fat variety (~1-1.5%). Go for the paper (tetrapack) containers which will protect milk from light, thus helping to retain its valuable vitamins.
The same goes for yogurt: choose low-fat over fat free.

**Orange, grapefruit juice**
Select the kind of juice that is not made from concentrate and has pulp.
I recommend getting the actual oranges (or other citruses) and squeeze their juices fresh.
Great for the mornings!

**Salad dressings**
Vinaigrettes made with olive oil are probably your healthiest bottled-dressing options out there.
Thin them with yogurt, milk, mild rice vinegar, or even (herb) tea to make them last longer! This little trick will also help you consume fewer calories.
Toss your salad with dressing right before serving. You will be using less this way.

## Mayonnaise, ketchup

You either make them or don't eat them, unless you know they come from a reputable non-factory source. The ones we grew up with are all commercially available and factory made with a list of chemicals that you want to stay away from. The only exceptions maybe the bio-organic/organic varieties of these condiments, available in better grocery stores selling whole foods.

## A quick advice for storing «doggy bags» from restaurant visits:

Transfer the content of «doggy bags», take-outs and leftovers into microwave-safe containers as soon as you can. Never reheat it in the take-out trays or plastic containers that aren't specifically microwave-safe!

# STEP 3 - REARRANGE YOUR FOOD RESERVES

This usually means to keep your fridge and pantry or kitchen cabinets neat by grouping the belonging food items together!

This will help you store, find and keep restocking your foods in a much more efficient way! If you know where everything is you will always have a better sense of how much you have, how fresh it is and when you will need to refill your supply.

There are many ways you can do this depending on the shape and size of the available storage therefore there is no right or wrong way.

## How To Switch To Eating Clean

Here are few ideas for your fridge that may help you.

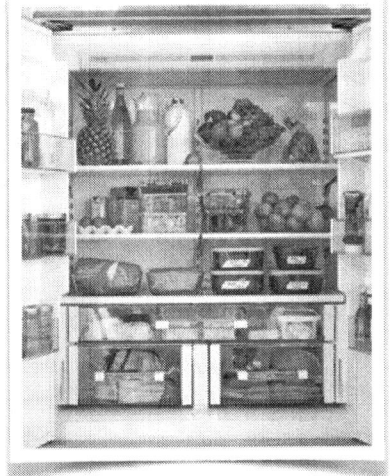
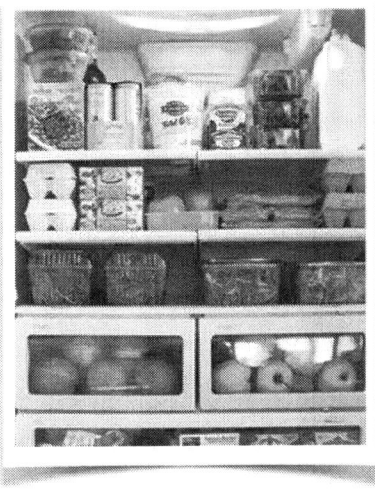
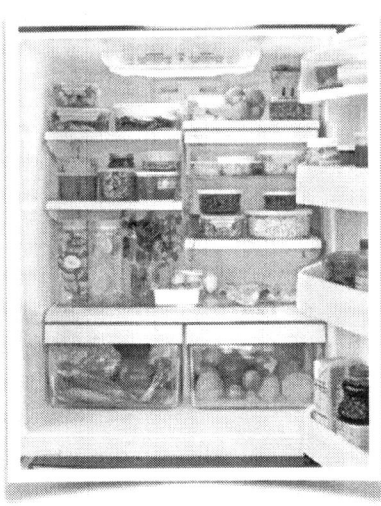
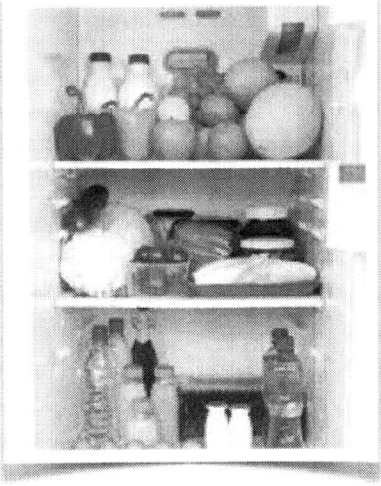

## How To Switch To Eating Clean

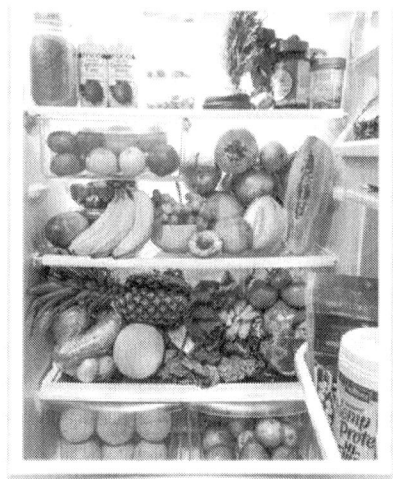
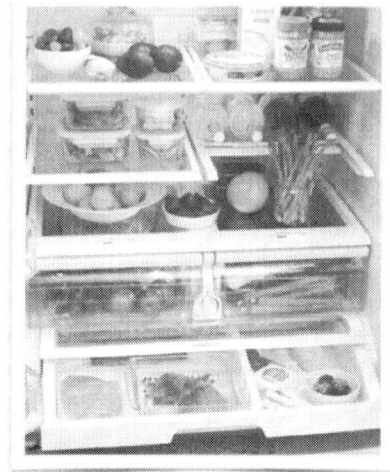
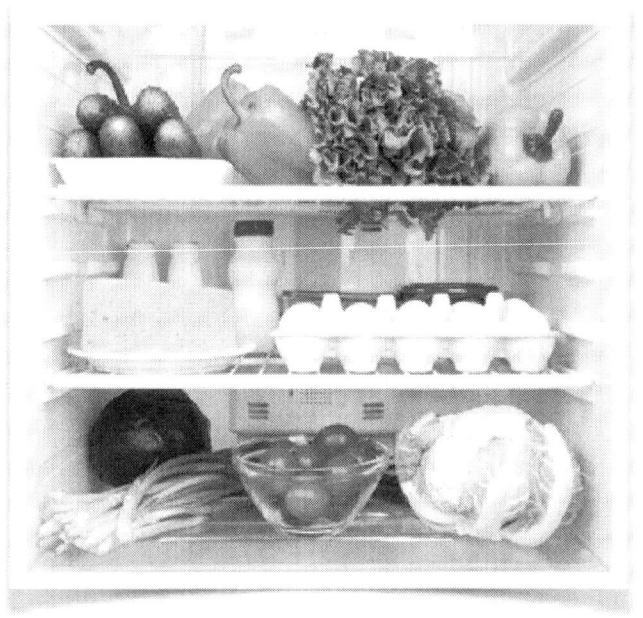

## The Importance of Balance

Did you know your body craves homeostasis? It means it wants to be in balance. This is not so good news for fad dieters because the more restrictive their diet is the stronger the yoyo effect will hit them. It is like a pendulum: it swings in one direction and reaches a maximum point where it stops for a moment. This tells you it will swing into the same maximum point on the other side, as a result of the primary swing. The same happens to your body when your weight loss diet is too long and too restrictive - it will swing back with a vengeance making you binge like it doesn't matter. This is how your body is trying to find its balance and it will find it whether you want it or not.

But let's see what happens when you eat clean consistently!

Our imaginary pendulum will slow down and ultimately stop swinging. It is predictable because extreme eating habits will add momentum to it and well-balanced eating habits along with eating clean will slowly kill its movement.

When you keep on eating clean foods your body will ultimately find a sort of "standstill" balance. This balance can be best described as a pendulum that doesn't swing. As stationary as it sounds, it is a good thing!

## Food Logistics

One of the key stones of eating clean is to have your choice of quality foods ready when you need them. Achieving this takes logistics. You don't have to be a master at it but you are very strongly recommended to have at least the basics down. When you eat clean, having fresh food is crucial so besides logistics you may want to be consistent not just on a daily, but also on a weekly basis. To always have a selection of clean foods available for you takes preparation. Besides getting the actual ingredients from different vendors and venues (a subject which we already touched) you will want to establish your own weekly schedule for certain times and days every week when you prep your foods. This can occur anywhere between daily to 2-3 times a week but not really less than that because the cleaner you eat the faster your food will spoil. So technically, if you want your food to be fresh and delicious when you eat it you know it shouldn't sit in your fridge for more than a day or two. Natural foods, if kept properly, may last even over a week but most of the fresh fruits, veggies, juices, raw milk only have about 24-48 hours before some decline in quality occurs. This decline is not necessarily very noticeable and definitely not something that will stop you from eating your food but since eating clean is all about eating quality foods I'd say freshness is a vital quality so I rather recommend doing your prep work a little more often than having to eat anything that might be even a bit subpar.

«What is it exactly that this food prepping entails?»
I'm glad you asked! This greatly depends on the type of food.

I tried to divide this section into food types although I realize this is not the only way you can do it.

## How To Switch To Eating Clean

## **VEGETABLES**

First and foremost, you will want to clean, cut and portion your veggies. Leafy greens can be rolled up and sliced into strips. Dry them in a salad centrifuge or between dry towels then distribute them into your favorite plastic boxes and into the fridge with them! If you make sure they are not overly wet and don't put any dressing or sauce on them they will be good for the next 3-7 days, depending on the type of your vegetables.

## **FRUITS**

You can do the same with fruits! If it is anything with pits like plums, peaches or apricots wash them, cut them in half, get the pit out and slice them or dice them. When kept dry and stored properly in a container of your choice in the fridge they should be fine and ready to eat for a couple of days but this too greatly depends on the ripeness and the type of fruit.

If it is a fruit with inside fruit meat and with a perfect natural outside "wrapper" like banana or apples, I don't like to prep them. They are as perfect as they come. If you still must prep them for some reason I recommend not doing it more than a few hours before you plan on consuming them. These fruits oxidize fairly quickly. They get brown easily unless you store them in special airtight vacuum containers. Another trick to keep the likes of apples and bananas fresh and un-browned in a regular container is to shred them or pulpify them and sprinkle or mix the resulting mass with one of nature's best antioxidant: freshly squeezed lemon juice!
Surely, it will be a bit more sour than normal but your fruit meat will not oxidize!

Berries and other relatively tiny drop shaped fruits can be picked from their stems, store them in a regular container but only wash them directly before eating them! If you keep them washed, chances are, they may start going bad a lot sooner. If the type of berry is way too small to pick them without actually harming or squishing the little berries (like wild strawberries or some kinds of red currants) just simply don't prep them.

One of my favorite fruit prepping trick is with melons. Honeydew or watermelon - it doesn't matter. It works with all sorts of melons. Cut the melon in four quarters and cut approximately equally sized cubes out of the inside with a knife. Alternatively, you can use a spoon or a melon baller to carve out spheres. Put these in your favorite container with a lid and into the fridge with it! Chilled melon is really good!

The cool thing about this trick is that you can chill your melon a lot faster (because you don't waste time and energy on cooling the rind which is usually thick) besides melons represent an odd, space wasting type of shape in the fridge when they are whole. Store them in food containers and you will not need that much space.

Avocados too brown very easily so they require a special kind of fruit prepping method. It only requires a piece of Saran wrap and a regular rubber ring. The idea is, you only peel and slice as much of the avocado as you are ready to eat right away and you cover the freshly cut surface with the Saran wrap. Use the rubber band to keep it in place and as tight as possible then simply put it in the fridge.

Alternatively, you can make guacamole from the avocados, put it in an airtight vacuum container or if you use regular containers pour some olive oil on top to cut off air to the surface, then you can store it in your fridge. Stays fresh and green for about a day or two.

## How To Switch To Eating Clean

## **MEATS**

When you eat clean you may or may not want to eat meat but most clean eaters who are also meat eaters eat the lean type of meats like the white parts (breasts) of the chicken and turkey, or maybe lean ground beef or buffalo but nothing too greasy or heavy.
I hope it goes without saying that hotdogs, baloneys, salamis and other "factory made" cold cut type of foods are NOT meat! For your own well-being's sake, stay away from them!
I recommend storing your meats in a ready-to-serve state like the chicken breasts should be skinned, unboned, grilled and even sliced into strips or diced into cubes. Boy, does it come handy when you just quickly want to sprinkle your evening salads with a bit of extra protein!

If you are not into grilling or simply your situation doesn't allow it, buy a whole rotisserie chicken skin it, bone it and dissect it with your hands. Once you separated the meat from the bones just cut it up to your liking, put them in a regular container and off it goes into the fridge!

## **BREADS, GRAINS, FLOUR, CEREALS AND NUTS**

The only thing that I need to say about these that they should also be kept in your fridge!
These not only stay fresh when stored in your icebox, they also don't go rancid. Moths and other nasty fliers or crawlers don't have a chance to spoil your goods either. When you store some grains or nuts in a ground form it is absolutely vital to keep them in your fridge because they tend to go rancid a lot faster when they are ground. For maximum freshness store your ground grains or seeds (like ground flaxseed, poppy, sesame, etc.) in the freezer. If you do this, remember to consume them within 1-2 months.

## **EGGS, DAIRY**

Eggs are a great way to add some more valuable nutrients to your meals along with a dash of extra protein! You can make a batch of 10 minute hard boiled eggs but don't peel them! Keep them in their shells and put them back in their original paper egg container. If you keep them in the fridge like this, you know where to reach whenever you need a few slices of hard boiled egg for a sandwich or a few hard boiled eggs for a quick egg salad, or just grab one and crumble it on top of your evening salad!

Dairy products come in various forms and if you get them from your supermarket they probably come factory packaged. Most cheese comes wrapped, possibly sliced, shredded or otherwise prepared for consumption. In some places, usually at farmers' markets, you can buy raw milk products and the packaging may greatly vary.

Cheese is probably the only dairy product that may require some prep work like slicing or grating if you buy it in whole. The same rule applies here as with mostly anything you prep: when you slice, chop, cut, grate stuff you make its breathing surface larger. The bigger the surface the more it is exposed to the oxygen in the air so either

- cover the surface
- get the air out of the box
- consume your food as soon as possible, before it even has a chance to go stale or bad.

So slices or shreds of cheese can be safely kept in ziplock bags or containers. But I'm sure you already knew that.

## Tips & Tricks To Eating Clean

Besides eating quality, naturally nutritious foods there are a few ideas that can help you reach your full potential and propel you to the next level of healthy living.
The following principles are based on nutrition science and common sense. If properly applied they can make a huge difference in your health, energy level and appearance, as I said, beside the good, clean food you eat.

### Combinations

We all combine foods when we eat yet we do it based on outdated, possibly unhealthy traditions and most of us really don't even have the faintest idea what we are doing and end up combining whatever feels good to us but not necessarily what is good to our well-being.

Combining two or more types of foods may actually amplify or mute certain effects in your body. In other words, the mere simultaneous presence of certain biochemical substances in you may determine what your body will do and how it will react to them.
Certain foods do really well with others therefore exerting a powerful synergistic effect on your body. It could be what we consider good or bad. Some other food combinations only have a weak synergy together therefore their presence will not have a pronounced effect on your biochemistry.

The details of this phenomena are beyond the scope of this publication but discussed in my other book titled "4 Secrets of Eating Right". (Available soon on-line.)

### Portions

Portion control may be one of the most crucial aspects of eating healthy! In our time and day, we generally tend to overeat. As a matter of fact, overeating seems to be a widely accepted first world problem although the acceptable portions tend to differ from one culture to another. One of the worst statistics originate from the United States which should not be a surprise; just look at the sizes of US fast food portions and the sugary drinks that come with them!

The proper portion size is different for everyone. Determining it requires to take your weight, sex, age, metabolic rate, body type, body composition and many other related factors into consideration.
Although the scope of this publication is not this, the general rule of thumb regarding a proper portion size is simple; eat only as much as will make you feel "un-hungry" but not quite full. In classic nutritionist writings, this amount measures to a not very scientific "one and a half cupped handful" of food, assuming you eat high quality, nutritious food at least 5 times a day, 2-3 hours apart.
Here is the biomechanics of overeating:
When you eat more than you should the wall of your stomach will start stretching, thus making your stomach bigger. You will want to feel the same «fullness» at your next meal so you overeat again and the same thing will happen. So the evil cycle is: filling up more room requires eating more food. Eating more food makes your stomach bigger. Now there is even more room in your stomach to be filled! So you need more food… I am sure you can see a repeating cycle emerging here. This is the general cause for most bulging guts, if not necessarily the direct cause for excess body fat.

## Timing

Timing can also be responsible for a lot of good, if done right and a lot of misery, if done poorly. If you nail timing your meals then you start eating when you should and stop when you should, but it is not just when you eat but how often you eat.

## How To Switch To Eating Clean

If your meals are too close to each other, your metabolism may instantly pay the price; your digestion probably won't have enough time to fully process your meal before your next one, thus not being able to digest to its full potential. If it is the other way around and your meals are too far apart, your blood sugar levels may dramatically drop so your brain won't be able to function properly, your body may go into emergency mode slowing down your metabolism wreaking havoc in your system.

## **The Four White Devils**

Another great and simple way (also a perfect first step towards eating clean) is to avoid the Four White Devils. Sometimes these are also referred to as the Four Horsemen of Fat-O-Calypse:
- White flour
- Sugar
- Animal fats and dairy
- Salt

While there is still a vehement debate going on whether which one of these substances, if any, are actually so harmful that you need to avoid them completely, I found it advisable to consume these with a lot of caution. It is good to be aware of what they can do to you in certain quantities, if eaten on a regular basis but leaving them behind altogether is also a great option, as the lack of them will not cause any damage to your body.

## Success Stories

Switching to eating clean is well known to have incredible ramifications in one's life!
I have experienced what it can do first hand, in my life, but I have also seen how it helped others even when all hope seemed to have gone.
Please read these stories and know that these aren't the only ones around but in my opinion these display the hidden healing power of eating clean robustly.
I changed the names of individuals to protect identities and preserve their privacy.

**The Story of N**
N has always been a naturally skinny little girl, then a skinny teenager and a skinny adult. Although being naturally skinny is what most people only dream about it isn't always a dream. N was born and raised in Eastern Europe so obviously she has been brought up with her Eastern European country's eating traditions, as for the everyday norm. Needless to say, these traditions are way outdated and nutritionally speaking disastrous. N felt it too as she had a bunch of medical conditions or better yet a rather huge collection of medical conditions that didn't disrupt her life but made it very inconvenient for her and sometimes even borderline unbearable.
These included an almost permanent migraine, a very unhealthy skin tone, huge, inflamed acnes on her back, cellulitis, extremely strong foot odor, warts on her hands, fungus on her feet, too much sweating, feminine problems (like irregular menstrual cycles, menstrual aches), hormonal problems, breast tension and super-sensitivity just to mention the worst ones.
The contrast is also interesting. A few short months after N transitioned to eating clean most of these issues seemed to have normalized and finally completely disappeared when N went all the way and minimized the animal originated foods in her diet. She ultimately became a

## How To Switch To Eating Clean

vegetarian, the kind who still eats fish, dairy and eggs - only no meat and her recent blood tests 14 years later are actually better than ever: her red blood cell count is perfect, minerals are way above normal, her white blood cell regulation is super and all of this is with a very healthy, naturally regulated low blood pressure.

Another interesting fact about N: she was already a clean eater vegetarian when she got pregnant with her first son M. The older, traditionally eating females in her family advised her to eat meat and heavy, greasy pork/potato based foods so she can have a healthy child. N, of course, refused to give in as she already knew the beneficial effects of eating clean. Nine months later she gave birth to a very healthy, strong boy, M. While N only had gained about 4 pounds in total during her pregnancy.

A further interesting fact is that her son M has always been eating very similarly to N despite the fact that bad, traditional eating habits were constantly present around them in their family yet they didn't seem to have been much of an influence, let alone temptation, to either of them. Interestingly, M says this kind of eating clean and healthy gives him an incredible amount of comfort that he can't really explain. This shouldn't come as a surprise as we know a pregnant mother shares almost all the nutrients in her blood stream with the fetus in her womb through the placenta. Recent studies suggest that our first memories form in our mother's womb. These early memories could be anything from sounds (like the mother's heartbeat) or just being in the fetus position or even «feeling» a certain way due to the given shared chemical balance. These memories seem to stay with us for the rest of our lives embedded deeply in the foundations of our psyche. If you connect these two bits of information you may have a hypothesis on your hands: if the baby's first memories are of the «healthy-chemistry» kind and they may link to feeling safe and loved, hence he will strive for it subconsciously or otherwise through the entirety of his life.

## How To Switch To Eating Clean

**The Story of V**
V was actually related to N. She was N's sister in law and was one of the family members that teased N and gave her a really hard time when she started her transition to eating clean as a vegetarian. It is but ironic that years after being as nasty to N as one can get V was diagnosed with a very serious case of rapidly worsening sclerosis multiplex. It crippled her quickly more and more day after day.
Desperately and unsuccessfully trying a series of modern medical approaches V was about to give up. By this time her sclerosis multiplex had advanced so much she was almost 100% wheelchair bound and in an incredible amount of pain.
Acting on N's advice, almost as a last resort, V consulted with a natural healer who recommended her a new lifestyle of eating clean, and in her case, a strictly organic raw vegan diet.
Shortly after entirely switching out her eating habits V's situation gradually became better until she seemed to have fully recovered without any leftover symptoms.
Now, it is debatable whether her full recovery was due to eating clean or the actual strict organic raw vegan diet but I'd say it was the mixture of both and it being organic had the main role. You may follow a raw vegan diet but you may still want to eat as clean as possible for best results; you just can't get around eating quality foods if you want to eat clean. Either way, V's story is a true testament to what difference your diet or your eating habits can make in your life.
Almost a decade after her seemingly fatal diagnosis, V is still gladly on her raw vegan regiment free of symptoms: she studies languages, regularly takes yoga classes and as productive, mobile and happy as one can get.

# How To Switch To Eating Clean

**The Story of C**

Now, C was a real wild child. A party animal from his early teen years, trying out everything and anything that could alter his mind and didn't care if it changed his body. This included alcohol, cigarettes and drugs of all sorts. So far away from being healthy, let alone being health conscious his focus was not at all on eating cleaner. He was really heavy, weighing about 220 lbs. Also he was visibly «puffed up» and undernourished at the same time. (Technically, a big, fat guy with skinny arms.) It was not until his mid twenties when he realized that he couldn't go on living like that. The sudden, surprising death of a few of his friends gave him the initial jolt to do a thorough self review. This is when he started to clean up his act: he quit doing drugs, drinking and even smoking. All within a year. Then he started focusing on living a healthier life. This included sweating at least three times a week for at least 30 minutes, drinking more filtered water and cutting out the crap food. Later the latter one changed to eating better quality foods.

He didn't have the help of a nutritionist because he couldn't afford one. He didn't have the internet's help either because this story is taking place in a pre-internet «for-information-go-to-the-library» kind of stone age era called the early nineties. It took C about 15 years to learn and figure out the basics of healthy nutrition and realize that the more you know the more you realize how much you still don't!

He is still learning today but he is relatively more knowledgeable than most people so he actually counts as one of the leading authorities in this regard.

Yes, it is my story. I am C.

## In Closing

I hope this friendly packet of condensed information was helpful to you and this publication was able to give you some value along with my personal gift to you: the FREE AUDIO BOOK VERSION of this book!
If you haven't yet gotten it, you can grab it here:
http://eatingclean.kormarton.com/

**If you enjoyed this book please leave a review on amazon.com!**

Should you have any feedback, questions, ideas, recommendations or criticism - I'd be happy to hear from you!
I'd like to make this book the ultimate authority in switching to eating clean so any help from you is greatly appreciated as I will update this eBook from time to time if and when new information comes to my attention!

Please visit my website, be my friend on Facebook, follow me on Twitter and subscribe to me on Youtube!
https://www.facebook.com/KorMartonWeightLoss
https://www.youtube.com/channel/UCgMM7v_IBK-zFn0ZQ8hxraQ
https://twitter.com/KorMarton
Thank you again for reading this book and good luck with your journey!

Copyright © 2016 by Kor Marton

All rights reserved. No part of this publication may be reproduced, distributed, or transmitted in any form or by any means, including photocopying, recording, or other electronic or mechanical methods, without the prior written permission of the publisher, except in the case of brief quotations embodied in critical reviews and certain other noncommercial uses permitted by copyright law. For permission requests, write to the publisher, addressed "Attention: Permissions Coordinator," at the address below.

Planetkor Publishing
18375 Ventura Blvd #379
Tarzana, CA 91356
www.planetkor.com

Kor@planetkor.com

First Edition

Made in the USA
Lexington, KY
05 January 2017